AF687677

I Still Live

McDougal & Associates

Servants of Christ and Stewards of the Mysteries of God

I Still Live

A 52-WEEK DEVOTIONAL FOR THOSE WHO ARE TRAVELING THE LONG, UNFORGIVING ROAD CALLED *CANCER*

by

Carolyn Brock

I STILL LIVE

Published by:

McDougal & Associates
18896 Greenwell Springs Road
Greenwell Springs, LA 70739
www.thepublishedword.com

McDougal & Associates is dedicated to the spreading of the Gospel of Jesus Christ to as many people as possible in the shortest time possible.

ISBN 978-1-940461-31-1

Printed in the US, the UK and Australia
For Worldwide Distribution

Dedication

I dedicate this book to my mother, who faithfully prays for me every single day.

Acknowledgements

I must thank my son, daughter, son-in-law, grandchildren and friends for their words of encouragement as I wrote the book during periods of severe suffering.

Contents

Do not be afraid, for I am with you.
Do not be discouraged, for I am your God.
I will strengthen you and help you.
I will hold you up with my victorious right hand. Isaiah 41:10

Introduction

(My Story)

In March of 2009, life started hitting me with some very hard blows. I was at work one day and developed what I thought was heartburn. I drank some hot tea, and the pain went away. Each time the discomfort returned, I drank some more tea. I finished my day of work, drove home and drank another cup of tea before going to bed.

During the night I was awakened with what felt like a sword going into the middle of my chest. I was rushed to the Emergency Room by ambulance and found myself lying on a stretcher in the Cardiac Catheter Lab. I had suffered a severe heart attack involving a 100% occlusion of the LAD (an important artery that feeds the heart muscle). I should have died, I was told. The occlusion of this artery is widely known in the medical industry as "the widow maker." Many people do not survive it. They placed a stent in that artery, and *I Still Live.*

By March of 2011 I had been experiencing bloating after eating for a couple of months. Then my abdomen started enlarging until it looked as if I was pregnant. Concerned, my daughter took me to the Emergency Room. After several tests, I was diagnosed with stage 3 metastatic primary peritoneal cancer, stemming from ovarian cancer. The fluid was removed from my abdomen, and I was given five months to live.

I underwent extensive abdominal surgery and was placed on a regimen of chemotherapy. A week after the first dose, I was scheduled for laboratory work, to ensure that the medication had not lowered my white blood cell count, my hemoglobin and hematocrit, my platelets and several electrolytes. These are very common side effects of chemotherapy. The low counts can be deadly if not caught in time.

The day I was scheduled for the blood tests I decided to do some grocery shopping before going to the hospital. When I walked into the grocery store at nine o'clock in the morning, there were no customers in the facility. Usually the store is very busy at that time. I asked if the store was open to customers. The staff assured me that it was. They were passing the time by washing all the surfaces of the checkout areas with bleach wipes.

After shopping I went to the hospital and had my blood drawn. An hour after arriving home, I received a phone call from the hospital. They warned me not to go out to public areas because my white blood cell count was very low, and I was in danger of catching any diseases I came into contact with. I then understood why the store had been empty and the staff had been wiping surfaces down with bleach wipes. God had gone before me to protect me. Although I did not know what to expect from this cancer journey, I knew without a doubt that He was going before me and preparing my way.

I began suffering other side effects from the chemotherapy. The fatigue was intolerable. I slept all day. The neuropathy in my hands and feet was disabling. My gait became unsteady, and I had to start using a cane when I walked. I awoke to nausea every morning.

I lost all my hair. I developed sores in my mouth. My short-term memory was failing me. My eyesight deteriorated, and I lost the ability to drive at night. Sometimes I felt like I was dying, and I pleaded with God, and He gave me the strength and will to live. In August of that year I went into remission, and I was sure that the journey was over for me.

Another March arrived, this one in 2012, and the cancer returned. I was placed on another regimen of chemo. In August I developed a severe headache. I was rushed to the Emergency Room by ambulance. By the time I arrived I was having stroke symptoms. Tests revealed that I had developed an intracranial hemorrhage that involved nearly half of my brain. This was brought on by the chemotherapy. I was not expected to survive based on my stroke symptoms and test results.

Plans were made to perform brain surgery, if needed, to remove the clot, but surgery was never required. The clot gradually decreased in size, as my body absorbed it. God continued to show Himself faithful, and I continued to live.

I went into remission again ... until March of 2013. Then the cancer returned with metastasis to my stomach, liver and spleen. I was, again, placed on a regimen of chemotherapy.

Before starting the chemotherapy, I required a MUGA (multigated acquisition) scan of my heart, to make sure it could tolerate the chemo. This specific chemotherapy was known to cause an enlarged heart, which could lead to congestive heart failure.

It was at this time that God put it on my heart to write this book. I was talking to Him about all the suffering I'd had to endure. He told me that I would comfort others, just as He had comforted me. When I asked Him what type of book I was to write, He spoke to my heart about a devotional for people diagnosed with cancer, just like me. In it, I could share my personal testimony.

When I asked God to show me how He wanted me to present the material, He first led me to a prayer from the Scriptures. I then developed a short devotional based on what I was experiencing with Him, the cancer and the chemotherapy. Then He gave me an encouraging word about the situation based on His promises and showed me that the devotionals should end with a confession of faith.

Each day I wrote the confession for that day on an index card and carried it with me all day in a pocket. I read it frequently throughout the day, to get God's Word into my heart. That also reminded me of the contents of the devotional throughout the day. As they developed, those devotionals turned into a book that could be used by others for encouragement as they traveled their own cancer journey.

I went into remission again in August of 2013. The MUGA scan was repeated, to see how much heart damage had occurred. Amazingly, my heart was now stronger than when I had started the chemotherapy. I laughed at this and praised God. It was His will that *I Still Live* and that the latter part of this journey be better than the first.

In January of 2014 the cancer again returned. This time I only had a short remission period. I was started on intravenous chemotherapy again and told I would never see remission again, that I only had three months before my quality of life was greatly diminished. I was also told that I would need Hospice intervention.

I was switched over to oral chemotherapy in July. I took it every day for twenty-one days, followed by a week off. This medication was the last treatment option for my case.

In December of 2014, I began having chest pain that mimicked the pain I had experienced with the heart attack. My cardiologist was concerned that the stented artery might be developing a blockage, and so he scheduled me for a cardiac catheterization the next day. The test was negative for any heart issues. The chemotherapy was causing the chest pain.

Next I became disoriented. I was unsure that I was on the right road when I went to the store. I thought my walk-in closet was my bathroom. I kept mixing up dates. I became very unsure of my ability to live alone. Upon sharing my symptoms with the cancer clinic, I was told the cancer had metastasized to my brain and that I would have to report to the Emergency Room of the university hospital immediately.

My daughter, son-in-law and I had to travel an hour from home to the hospital. This was the only hospital that had the resources available — in case I needed emergency brain surgery. We arrived at the hospital, and testing began immediately. All the results came back negative. In fact, there were no abnormal issues with my brain at all. Now I had even more for which to praise God.

In January of 2015 I was told that I had four months to live. If I stayed on the chemotherapy, the side effects of it would kill me, and if I stopped the chemotherapy, I still only had four months to live because the cancer would kill me. It has been a month, and *I Still Live* an abundant and satisfying life, and it is now time to publish this book.

It is my prayer that these devotionals encourage you on your journey, just as they have encouraged me as I wrote them. I praise God for His faithfulness. I thank Him for His mercy and love. I give Him all the glory that *I Still Live* four years into this journey. And I trust that He has my future in His loving hands.

Carolyn Brock
Raleigh, North Carolina

WEEK 1

The Beginning of the Journey

PRAYER:

Lord God, You keep track of all my sorrows. You have collected all my tears in Your bottle. You have recorded each one in Your book. I know You are on my side. I praise Your for Your promises. I trust in You. I will not be afraid.

In Jesus' name I pray.
Amen!

(based on Psalm 56:8-11)

DEVOTIONAL:

The beginning of my cancer journey was very difficult. I went to my first clinic appointment alone, not knowing what to expect. As I took a seat in the waiting room, I noticed all the signs on the walls contained the word *cancer*. All the books laid out for patients to read contained the word *cancer* in their titles. Everywhere I looked that word *cancer* shouted at me. The urge to cry suddenly overpowered me. I could not hold it back. I cried and cried and cried. I felt like I was making a scene as I sat alone crying in that room.

I was finally called into the exam room. I was still crying, and the nurse gave me permission to cry some more. That word *cancer* continued to yell at me. Reality set in: I HAD CANCER! I had no idea what to expect on this journey. I feared the suffering at the end.

A WORD FROM GOD:

The Lord watches over those who fear him,
those who rely on his unfailing love.
He rescues them from death
and keeps them alive in times of famine.
Put your hope in the Lord.
He is our help and our shield.

Psalm 33:18-20

CONFESSION OF FAITH:

I put my hope in the Lord. He is my Help and my Shield.

WEEK 2

You Are My God

PRAYER:

My Lord, You are my God. I am trusting in You. My future is in Your hands. Rescue me from the side effects of this chemotherapy. Let Your favor shine on Your servant. In Your unfailing love, rescue me. O Lord, I call out to You for help.

In Jesus' name I pray.
Amen!

(based on Psalm 31:14–17)

DEVOTIONAL:

This cancer journey is under God's control regardless of what it throws at us. He loves us and cares for us. Such knowledge enables us to remain steadfast in our faith in His ability to rescue us. It helps us wait patiently for Him to work out His timetable for our healing. He took our sicknesses and removed our diseases (see Isaiah 53:4) when He died on the cross and rose again. It is finished. We just need to wait patiently to see God's Word manifest itself in our bodies.

A WORD FROM GOD:

Give your burdens to the LORD,
and he will take care of you.
He will not permit the godly to slip and fall.
Psalm 55:22

CONFESSION OF FAITH:

As I give my burdens to the LORD, He takes care of me.

WEEK 3

God Is Faithful to His Promises

PRAYER:

Father, I hold tightly to Your Word without wavering. I know You can be trusted to keep Your promises.

In Jesus' name I pray.
Amen!

(based on Hebrews 10:23)

DEVOTIONAL:

The Scriptures give us hope and encouragement as we wait patiently for God's promises to be fulfilled (see Romans 15:4). Knowledge of them affects how we respond to our suffering, today and in the future.

Some Christian denominations deny that healing is part of the New Testament, but Jesus told us otherwise. A man with leprosy knelt before Him and said, *"If you are willing, you can heal me and make me clean."* Jesus reached out and touched him. *"I am willing,"* He said, *"Be healed!"* And instantly the leprosy disappeared (Matthew 8:2-3). Jesus said that it was His will that we be healed and made whole and complete. He purchased our healing with His own blood. Peter wrote to the first-century church:

By his wounds I am healed. 1 Peter 2:24

We must ask the Father for our healing because we are unable to heal ourselves. Jesus came to do the Father's will, not His own (see John 6:38). The Father put Jesus into a healing ministry. Jesus obeyed and went about healing people. Since the Father put Jesus into a healing ministry, we know that it is also His will that we be healed. Furthermore, the Bible gives us God's promises regarding our healing.

HEALING PROMISES:

Daughter, be encouraged! Your faith has made you well. Matthew 9:22

Because of your faith it will happen.
Matthew 9:29

Daughter, your faith has made you well. Go in peace. Your suffering is over. Mark 5:34

The LORD forgives all my sins, and heals all my diseases. Psalm 103:3

He sent out his Word and healed them, snatching them from the door of death.
Psalm 107:20

I am the LORD who heals you. Exodus 15:26

O LORD, if you heal me I will be truly healed.
Jeremiah 17:14

For you who fear my name, the Sun of Righteousness will rise with healing in his wings. And you will go free, leaping with joy like calves let out to pasture. Malachi 4:2

LORD, you restore my health and allow me to live! You have rescued me from death and forgiven all my sins. Isaiah 38:16-17

"I will give you back your health and heal your wounds," says the LORD. Jeremiah 30:17

Believe that God keeps His promises despite your symptoms. Abraham was a hundred years old, and he figured that his body was as good as dead. Sarah was also barren. They both waited for the promise of a child despite their symptoms, and the result was that Isaac was born.

Do not waver in believing God's promises. Be fully convinced that He is able to do whatever He has promised.

A WORD FROM GOD:

The LORD always keeps his promises; he is gracious in all He does. Psalm 145:13

He keeps every promise forever. Psalm 146:6

CONFESSION OF FAITH:

The LORD always keeps His promises. He is gracious in all He does. He keeps every promise forever.

WEEK 4

I Do Not Fear Death

PRAYER:

LORD God, You will not leave my soul among the dead or allow me to rot in the grave. You will show me the way of life, granting me the joy of Your presence and the pleasures of living with You forever.

(based on Psalm 16:10-11)

DEVOTIONAL:

Since I am a child of God, I have the confidence that God will not forget me when I die. Death is not a dark door at the end of my life. For a child of God, death is a bright pathway to a new and better life — the doorway into eternal life. I do not fear death because I know God will bring me to life again, to live with Him forever.

You can have this same assurance. Salvation is not a complicated process.

For everyone has sinned; we all fall short of God's glorious standard. Romans 3:23

Consequently, we are all sinners, and sin cuts us off from our holy God. But all your sins can be forgiven, whether they are big or small.

The wages of sin is death, but the free gift of God is eternal life through Christ Jesus our Lord. Romans 6:23

Salvation is not something we earn because of some good we have done. It is a gift from God. He gives it to us because of His mercy and love.

God showed his great love for us by sending Christ to die for us while we were still sinners. Romans 5:8

God did not send Jesus to die for us because we were good enough, but because He loved us so much.

If you have not yet turned to Him, He still loves you.

> *If you confess with your mouth that Jesus is Lord and believe in your heart that God raised him from the dead, you will be saved. For it is by believing in your heart that you are made right with God, and it is confessing with your mouth that you are saved.* Romans 10:9-10

If you believe in your heart and say with your mouth that Jesus Christ is the risen LORD, you will be saved.

PRAYER OF SALVATION:

Dear LORD, I confess that I am a sinner and that I have come short of Your glory. But I believe that You love me and that Jesus died on the cross for my sins. I confess with my mouth that Jesus is LORD, and I believe in my heart that You have raised Him from the dead. I now receive Your wonderful gift of salvation through Jesus Christ my LORD, and I ask You to fill me with Your Holy Spirit.

In Jesus' name I pray.
Amen!

A WORD FROM GOD:

But to all who believe him [Jesus] and accept him [Jesus], he gives the right to become children of God. They are reborn — not with a physical birth resulting from human passion or plan, but a birth that comes from God.

John 1:12-13

See how very much our Father loves us, for he calls us his children, and that is what we are.

1 John 3:1

If you prayed the prayer of salvation, you are now a child of God, and you can have the confidence that God will not forget you when you die. Death is not a dark door at the end of your life. For a child of God, it is a bright pathway to a new and better life — the doorway into eternal life. Do not fear death, but know that God will bring you to life again, to live with Him forever.

CONFESSION OF FAITH:

I confess that Jesus is Lord and believe in my heart that God raised Him from the dead. I am now a child of God.

WEEK 5

Pray for Your Healing

PRAYER:

Father, the devil has wounded my body with cancer and the side effects of chemotherapy. Today — at this moment — I break the power of the devil over my body, and I claim my deliverance and healing in Jesus' name.

Your Word says I am healed. My doctors and other people around me tell me that I am dying from the chemotherapy and the cancer. But the matter is settled, and this prayer has been answered.

The Scriptures say I am healed, and the Scriptures do not lie because God cannot lie. Therefore I believe I am healed, even though I have not seen the healing manifested in my body.

Father, I thank You that I am healed. I praise You for my healing. I believe You are my Healer, just as You told me in Your Word.

In Jesus' name,
Amen!

DEVOTIONAL:

Personal prayer is very important when one is traveling the cancer journey. There is a process to follow. First, decide what you want from God. Then find the scriptures that promise you those things. It is these promises that assure you that your desire is God's will. If you cannot find scriptures to support your prayer, then you are outside of God's will, and you cannot expect the prayer to be answered.

Once you have your promises, meditate on them, to get them fixed in your spirit. God's Word tells us:

> *Study this Book of Instruction continually. Meditate on it day and night, so you will be sure to obey everything written in it. Only then will you prosper and succeed in all you do.* Joshua 1:8

The devil will try to make you doubt God so that he can rob you of your answer to the prayer.

But once God's promises are established in your spirit, you will always have an answer for the demons who will try to rob you of the answer to your prayer.

When the devil tempted Jesus in the wilderness, He rebuked him saying, *"No! The scriptures say, '…' "* (Matthew 4:4, 7 and 10), and He quoted the Word of God that was appropriate for the situation.

Sometimes we are tempted to give up on situations that have not changed for many years. But God can change what seems unchangeable and give us new purpose and hope. Those who suffer will mature under the hardship and have a deeper understanding of God's love.

God has given His promises regarding prayer. He tells us to ask Him for what we want and to believe that we receive it.

> *ASK THE FATHER directly, and He will grant your request because you USE MY [Jesus'] NAME. … Ask USING MY NAME, and you will receive, and you will have abundant joy.* John 16:23-24, Emphasis Mine

> *Have faith in God. I tell you the truth, you can say to this mountain "May you be*

lifted up and thrown into the sea; and it will happen. But YOU MUST BELIEVE IT WILL REALLY HAPPEN AND HAVE NO DOUBT IN YOUR HEART. I tell you, you can pray for anything, and if you believe you have received it, it will be yours. But when you are praying, first forgive anyone you are holding a grudge against, so that your Father in heaven will forgive you your sins, too.

Mark 11:22-25, Emphasis Mine

Again, be sure to have the Word of God to back up your prayer.

Finally, give thanks for everything to God the Father in the name of our Lord Jesus Christ.

Ephesians 5:20

A WORD FROM GOD:

My child, pay attention to what I say. Listen carefully to my words. Do not lose sight of them, let them penetrate deep into your heart, for they bring life to those who find them and healing to their whole body. Proverbs 4:20-22

Do not be impressed with your own wisdom. Instead, fear the LORD and turn away from evil. Then you will have healing for your body and strength for your bones.

Proverbs 3:7-8

CONFESSION OF FAITH:

I AM HEALED IN JESUS' NAME!

WEEK 6

I Believe

PRAYER:

O LORD, You are a great and awesome God! You always fulfill Your covenant and keep Your promises of unfailing love to those who love You and obey Your commands. You, LORD, are merciful and forgiving, even though we have rebelled against You.

(based on Daniel 9:4 and 9)

DEVOTIONAL:

It is our belief in Jesus that makes us right with God. Our faith is the inner confidence that He is who He says He is and that He is faithful to do what He says He will do.

Sometimes people respond to God's offer of healing with scoffing. It seems too simple, and they cannot accept the simple cure of faith. We need to humbly accept God's mercy. Our reaction to the way of faith can keep us from the cure we need the most.

A WORD FROM GOD:

The thief's [devil's] purpose is to steal, and kill and destroy. My [Jesus'] purpose is to give you a rich and satisfying life. John 10:10

CONFESSION OF FAITH:

I believe that by Jesus' wounds I am healed and will live a rich and satisfying life.

WEEK 7

I Choose to Live

PRAYER:

O Lord, I thank You for the favor You have shown me. In Your unfailing love, You have answered my prayer with Your sure salvation. You rescued me from the mud and did not let me sink deeper. You saved me from my enemies — cancer and chemotherapy — and pulled me from the deep waters of anguish. You did not let the floods overwhelm me, the deep waters swallow me or the pit of death devour me.

In Jesus' name I pray,
Amen!

DEVOTIONAL:

It would be easy to give up fighting cancer and the side effects of chemotherapy, but I choose not to die. Instead, I will live to tell what the LORD has done for me. It has been a difficult battle, but I still trust in God's sovereignty over my enemies. Because of His faithfulness, *I Still Live* to tell the story He has woven into my life.

A WORD FROM GOD:

... You are meant for better things, things that come with salvation. For God is not unjust. He will not forget how hard you have worked for him and how you have shown your love to him by caring for other believers, as you still do. Keep on loving others as long as life lasts, in order to make certain that what you hope for will come true. Then you will not become spiritually dull and indifferent. Instead, you will follow the example of those who are going to inherit God's promises because of their faith and endurance. Hebrews 6:9-12

CONFESSION OF FAITH:

I will not die; instead, I will live to tell what the LORD has done. Psalm 118:17

WEEK 8

The Loneliness of Cancer

PRAYER:

O Sovereign LORD, You have only begun to show Your goodness and the strength of Your hand to me, Your servant. Is there any god in Heaven or on Earth who can perform such great and mighty deeds as You do? My heart rejoices in You, LORD! You have made me strong. Now I have an answer for my enemies — chemotherapy and cancer.

I rejoice because You rescued me.
No one is holy like the LORD!
There is no one besides You;
there is no rock like our God. 1 Samuel 2:1-2

Please show them all Your glory, LORD, and extend my life by many years.

In Jesus' name I pray,
Amen!

DEVOTIONAL:

A life of cancer can be intensely lonely. Precious is that friend who steps in when loneliness tries to darken a day. A friend eases the loneliness. But God alone can satisfy our deepest longings. During sleepless, uncomfortable nights, meditate on all the ways God has already helped you. Let His blessings remind you that you are not alone. Greet each new day with songs of praise, and let God wrap you in His presence.

Be confident of God's control over the events of your life. Be thankful for all the blessings He has showered upon you.

A WORD FROM GOD:

Trust in the LORD and do good.
Then you will live safely in the land and prosper.
Take delight in the LORD,
and he will give you your heart's desires.

Commit everything you do to the LORD.
Trust him, and he will help you.
He will make your innocence radiate like the dawn,
and the justice of your cause will shine like the noonday sun.
Be still in the presence of the LORD,
and wait patiently for him to act.

Psalm 37:3-7

CONFESSION OF FAITH:

I rejoice because God is with me.

WEEK 9

Call on God in Your Loneliness

PRAYER:

O LORD, my God, *"my heart has heard you say, 'Come and talk with me.' And my heart responds, 'LORD, I am coming' "* (Psalm 27:8). I continually search for more of You and more of Your strength.

The heavens proclaim Your glory, O Sovereign LORD. The skies display Your craftsmanship. Day after day they continue to speak. Night after night they make You known. LORD God, please give me complete knowledge of Your will. Give me spiritual wisdom and understanding. I want my life to honor and please You and produce every kind of good fruit.

I deeply desire to know You better and better. Please strengthen me with all Your glorious power so that I will have all the endurance and patience I need.

Thank You for rescuing me from the kingdom of darkness and transferring me into the kingdom of Your dear Son, who purchased my freedom and forgave my sins.

In Jesus' name I pray,
Amen!

DEVOTIONAL:

You can call upon the LORD at any time, not just when troubles arise, but also to share your joy with Him when He blesses you. He loves the sound of your voice, and He is never far away.

Ask God to give you complete knowledge of His will and to give you spiritual wisdom and understanding, so that the way you live will always honor and please Him, and your life will produce every kind of good fruit. All the while, you will grow as you learn to know God better and better.

Pray that you will be strengthened with all His glorious power so you will have all the endurance and patience you need. May you be filled with joy, always thanking the Father. He has enabled you to share in the inheritance that belongs to His people, who live in the light. For He has rescued you from the kingdom of darkness and transferred you into the kingdom of His dear Son, who purchased your freedom and forgave your sins.

(based on Colossians 1:9-14)

A WORD FROM GOD:

Search for the LORD, and for his strength; continually seek him. 1 Chronicles 16:11

Darkness as black as night covers the nations of the earth, but the glory of the LORD rises and appears over you. Isaiah 60:2

CONFESSION OF FAITH:

God has enabled me to share in the inheritance that belongs to His people, who live in the light. God has rescued me from the kingdom of darkness and transferred me into the kingdom of His dear Son, who purchased my freedom and forgave my sins.

WEEK 10

You Are Never Alone

PRAYER:

O Lord, You have examined my heart and know everything about me. You know when I sit down or stand up. You know my thoughts even when I am far away. You see me when I travel and when I rest at home. You know everything I do. You know what I am going to say even before I say it, Lord.

You go before me and follow me. You place Your hand of blessing on my head. Such knowledge is too wonderful for me, too great for me to understand! I can never escape from Your Spirit! I can never get away from Your presence!

If I go up to Heaven, You are there. If I go down to the grave, You are there. If I ride the wings of the morning, if I dwell by the farthest oceans, even there Your hand will guide me, and

Your strength will support me. Thank You for Your devotion toward me, LORD God.

Amen!

(based on Psalm 139:1-10)

DEVOTIONAL:

Cancer can be a lonely existence. No one can really understand what we are going through ... unless they have been through it themselves. But God knows everything about us. Even though we have cancer, He still accepts and loves us. And if we let Him, He will wrap His arms more tightly around us.

He never leaves us. His presence if ever surrounding us, comforting us with His peace. He sees every tear we shed in the privacy of our rooms. He hears our questioning thoughts as we try to understand why we even have this disease.

He hovers over us when we are too fatigued to stay awake. His hand guides us, and His strength supports us when we fight the fatigue and conquer the tasks that need to be done.

He calms us when we become angry at life. He lifts us up when depression tries to bring us down. He supports us when we are too weak to take another step. In every situation that we go through, He is there, protecting, loving and guiding us. There is no greater love. He is never too far from us to help us, and cancer cannot isolate us from God's loving presence.

A WORD FROM GOD:

For the LORD your God is living among you.
He is a mighty savior.
He will take delight in you with gladness.
With his love he will calm all your fears.
He will rejoice over you with joyful songs .

Zephaniah 3:17

I will never fail you. I will never abandon you.

Hebrews 13:5

CONFESSION OF FAITH:

My God will never fail me. My God will never abandon me.

WEEK 11

Cancer Cannot Separate Me from the Love of God

PRAYER:

I pray that from His glorious and unlimited resources He will empower you with inner strength through His Spirit. Christ, please make Your home in their hearts as they trust in You. Make their roots grow down into Your love, and keep them strong. Give them the power to understand how wide, how long, how high and how deep Your love is. And may they experience the love of Christ, though it is too great to understand fully. Then they will be made complete with all the fullness of life and power that comes from You.

In Jesus' name I pray,
Amen!

(based on Ephesians 3:16-19)

DEVOTIONAL:

Because of Christ and our faith in Him, we can now come boldly and confidently into God's presence. When I think of this, I fall to my knees and pray to the Father, the Creator of everything in Heaven and on Earth (see Ephesians 3:12-15).

Can anything ever separate us from Christ's love? Does it mean He no longer loves us, if we have trouble or calamity, or are persecuted, or hungry, or destitute, or in danger, or threatened with death? (As the Scriptures say, "For your sake we are killed every day; we are being slaughtered like sheep.) No, despite all these things, overwhelming victory is ours through Christ, who loved us.

And I am convinced that nothing can ever separate us from God's love. Neither death nor life, neither angels or demons, neither our fears for today nor our worries about tomorrow — not even the powers of Hell can separate us from God's love. No power in the sky above or in the earth below — indeed, nothing in all creation will ever be able to separate us from the love of God that is revealed in Christ Jesus our L*ORD* . Romans 8:35-39

Nothing we suffer can compare to the great price Jesus paid to save us.

A WORD FROM GOD:

Since we are God's children, we are his heirs. In fact, together with Christ we are heirs of God's glory. But if we are to share his glory, we must also share his suffering.

Romans 8:17

CONFESSION OF FAITH:

I am convinced that nothing can ever separate me from God's love.

WEEK 12

Trust in the Lord's Unfailing Love

PRAYER:

O LORD, I give my life to You. I trust in You, my God! No one who trusts in You will ever be disgraced. Lead me by Your truth, for You are the God who saves me. All day long I put my hope in You. Remember, O LORD, Your compassion and unfailing love. Do not remember the rebellious sins of my youth. Remember me in the light of Your unfailing love, for You are merciful, O LORD.

In Jesus' name I pray,
Amen!

(based on Psalm 25:1-7)

DEVOTIONAL:

I take great delight in my LORD and experience great joy and pleasure in His presence. To do this, I must know Him because knowledge of His great love fills me with delight. I commit myself to Him and entrust everything to His control and guidance: my life, my family, my job, my possessions, my health, my finances. I trust that He can take care of me better than I can take care of myself. I am willing to wait patiently for Him to work out what is best for me. Many people think living for the LORD is futile, but I know His unfailing love will triumph over this cancer.

A WORD FROM GOD:

Trust in the LORD and do good.
Then you will live safely in the land and prosper.
Take delight in the LORD,
and he will give you your heart's desires.
Commit everything you do to the LORD.
Trust him and he will help you.
He will make your innocence radiate like the dawn,
and the justice of your cause will shine like the noonday sun.

Be still in the presence of the LORD,
and wait patiently for him to act.

Psalm 37:3-7

CONFESSION OF FAITH:

I will be still in the presence of the LORD, and wait patiently for Him to act.

WEEK 13

Cancer Cannot Come Between You and God

PRAYER:

Great and marvelous are Your works, O Lord God Almighty. Just and true are Your ways, O King of the nations. Who will not fear You, Lord, and glorify Your name? For You alone are holy. All nations will come and worship before You, for Your righteous deeds have been revealed.

Amen!

(based on Revelation 16:3-4)

DEVOTIONAL:

You have not been abandoned by Christ because you have cancer. It is impossible to be separated from His presence. Jesus, through His sacrifice on the cross, has already defeated this cancer with His blood. Because of God's great love, we can always feel totally secure in Him.

A WORD FROM GOD:

Know that the Son of God has come, and he has given you understanding so that you can know the true God. ... Live in fellowship with his Son, Jesus Christ. He is the only true God, and he is eternal life. 1 John 5:20

CONFESSION OF FAITH:

I have defeated Satan by the blood of the Lamb and by the word of my testimony (see Revelation 12:11).

WEEK 14

Chemotherapy Has Wounded My Body

PRAYER:

Lord God, chemotherapy has reduced my quality of life. I have grown weary in this present body, and I long to put on my heavenly body, like new clothing. For we will put on heavenly bodies. We will not be spirits without bodies.

While I live in this earthly body, I groan and sigh, but it is not that I want to die and get rid of this body that clothes me. Rather, I want to put on my new body so that this dying body will be swallowed up by life. You Yourself have prepared me for this and, as a guarantee, You have given me Your Holy Spirit.

O Lord, if You heal me, I will be truly healed. If You save me, I will be truly saved. My praises are for You alone. Come with great power, O God, and rescue me! Defend me with Your might. Listen to my prayer, O God. Pay attention to my plea. For chemotherapy is attacking me. Cancer is trying to kill me. They care nothing for You. But You are my Helper. You keep me alive! May the evil plans of the enemy be turned against him. Do as You promised and put an end to this suffering.

In Jesus' name I pray,
Amen!

(based on 2 Corinthians 5:2-10,
Jeremiah 17:14 and Psalm 54:1-5)

DEVOTIONAL:

My eyesight has failed. Chemo already led to a cataract removal once, and now it has affected the cataract in the other eye. Since I have visual difficulties at night, all my activities have to take place before the sun sets. Otherwise, I am dependent upon others to get me to and from destinations.

My short-term memory is failing me. I drive and forget where I am going. I go downstairs to do an errand and forget what I was going to do. I do my devotions and cannot remember them once I close the book. One day runs into the next, and I cannot remember the day or date.

My endurance is poor. I become short of breath, and my heart races with exertion. Fatigue overwhelms me.

My abdomen becomes extremely distended and painful when I eat, so that food has become my enemy, and going out to eat causes me great anxiety. My abdomen fills up with fluid that has to be removed with a needle. I have lost control of my bladder and bowels and worry about putting myself to shame in public.

My mouth becomes full of sores. All day long I walk around filled with grief. My health is broken. I am exhausted and completely crushed. My groans come from an anguished heart. My loved ones and friends stay away, fearing my disease. Even my own family stands at a distance. Meanwhile, chemotherapy and cancer lay traps to kill me (see Psalm 38:6-12).

A WORD FROM GOD:

I will restore you so you can continue to serve me. Jeremiah 15:19

I will give you back your health and heal your wounds. Jeremiah 30:17

He sent out his word and healed them, snatching them from the door of death.

Psalm 107:20

He [Jesus] was pierced for our rebellion,
crushed for our sins.
He [Jesus] was beaten so we could be whole;
He [Jesus] was whipped so we could be healed.

Isaiah 53:5

He [Jesus] personally carried our sins
in his body on the cross
so that we could be dead to sin
and live for what is right.
By his wounds
you are healed.

1 Peter 2:24

CONFESSION OF FAITH:

Jesus was pierced for my rebellion and crushed for my sins. He was beaten so I could be whole and whipped so I could be healed. By His wounds I am healed.

WEEK 15

Help this Agony in My Bones and Joints

PRAYER:

O Lord, My life is poured out like water, and all my bones are out of joint. At night my bones are filled with pain which gnaws at me relentlessly. Have compassion on me, Lord, for I am weak. Heal me, Lord, for my bones are in agony.

In Jesus' name I pray,
Amen!

(based on Psalm 22:14, Job 30:17 and Psalm 6:2)

DEVOTIONAL:

Chemotherapy has attacked my hands, feet, bones and joints. It feels like my toes and fingers are plugged into an electrical socket, which is sending electrical currents through my hands and feet. Walking without a cane is now unsafe for me since I cannot feel when my toes are on solid ground, due to this chemo-induced neuropathy. I feel like I have stones in the balls of my feet, and walking causes me great discomfort.

My knee and hip joints become very painful when I try to walk up and down the stairs in my home. Sometimes my knees buckle and I nearly fall.

When I try to sleep, the sheets cause my toes to burn. I develop cramps in my feet and calves at night. When I rise from the bed and stand, the pain attacks the long bones in both my lower legs. I find myself totally unable to walk because of the extreme pain.

I am sick at heart. How long, O Lord, until You restore me?

A WORD FROM GOD:

The Lord hears his people when they call to him for help.
He rescues them from all their troubles.
The Lord is close to the brokenhearted;
he rescues those whose spirits are crushed.
The righteous person faces many troubles,
but the Lord comes to the rescue each time.

For the LORD protects the bones of the righteous;
not one of them is broken.

Psalm 34:17-20

CONFESSION OF FAITH:

The LORD rescues me from all my troubles.

WEEK 16

Drawing on God's Strength

PRAYER:

O Lord God, in my feeble state, You give me power and strength. Although I am weak and tired and fall in exhaustion, I still trust You. As I trust, I find new strength. I walk and do not grow weary. You bring me to my feet. You give me the will to keep fighting this disease. Your power, O Lord, works best in my weakness. Please, Jesus, work Your power through me.

In Jesus' name I pray,
Amen!

(based on Isaiah 40:29–31)

DEVOTIONAL:

God never runs out of power and strength. You can always lean on Him when you become too feeble to carry on. He is never too busy to help you. He always has His ear turned toward you.

When you feel like life is crushing in on you, call upon Him to renew your strength. Patiently expect Him to fulfill His promises in His Word and to strengthen you enough to rise above life's difficulties.

Believe that He loves you and wants what is best for you. Confidently believe that He has the power to control all life — including yours. When your faith is struggling or weak, accept His provisions and care for you.

You can be courageous and hopeful when you are overcome with suffering. God can still use you. Let your limitations cause you to depend more upon Him for your effectiveness, instead of depending upon your own energy, effort or talent. When you admit your weaknesses and turn to God, you affirm that He has the strength to help you.

A WORD FROM GOD:

My grace is all you need. My power works best in weakness. 2 Corinthians 12:9-10

CONFESSION OF FAITH:

When I am weak, I trust in the Lord. Then I am strong.

WEEK 17

Never Give Up the Fight

PRAYER:

O Lord my God, I pray that from Your glorious, unlimited resources You will empower me with inner strength through Your Spirit. As I put my trust in You, make Your home in my heart, and my roots will grow down into Your love and keep me strong. And please give me the power to understand how wide, how long, how high and how deep Your love is for me. Let me experience the love of Christ so that I will be made complete with all the fullness of life and power that comes from You.

Thank You for redeeming and ransoming me and giving me the gift of eternal life. I have the peace of knowing that when You take me from this world, You will bring me into Your Kingdom and crown me with everlasting joy. There will be no more sorrow and mourning. I will be filled with joy and gladness. So, there is no fear of dying for me.

O LORD God, help me to run with endurance the race You have set before me. I will keep my eyes on Jesus, the Champion who initiates and perfects my faith. Because of the joy awaiting Him, He endured the cross, disregarding its shame. Now He is seated in the place of honor beside Your throne. Each time I become weak and think about giving up, remind me of all the hostility Jesus endured from sinful people and that I am running my race for Him.

In Jesus' name I pray,
Amen!

(based on Ephesians 3:16–19, Isaiah 35:8–10 and Hebrews 12:1–3)

DEVOTIONAL:

When we encounter suffering, it is easy to lose heart and quit. We start believing what all the unbelievers speak over us. "You will die from cancer," and "You will never be healed by God." Then they begin persecuting us for our faith, which adds to our suffering.

Instead of focusing on the suffering and persecution, as believers, we should consider the ultimate goal of standing in faith on God's Word. Athletes concentrate on the finish line and ignore their discomfort. As believers, we should focus on the reward for our faith rather than on our suffering.

Do not let your suffering (and the criticism you receive from others because of your faith) cause you to give up. Do not forsake your eternal reward because it becomes difficult listening to those who do not believe God's healing promises. There is good that can come out of your suffering. Let it remind you of how much Christ suffered for you to purchase your healing. Let it remind you to look beyond your brief life here.

No matter what happens in this life, we have the assurance of eternal life when all suffering and sorrow ends. There is a day coming when life will be peaceful. Allow the resurrection power of Christ to strengthen you throughout the day. As you journey through this terrible illness called *cancer,* remember that there is life after death.

As a believer, you will live forever in a place with God that contains no sin and suffering. As a believer you have eternal life ahead of you. Let it provide an opportunity for you to prove your faith to others. Your suffering provides an opportunity for God to demonstrate His power through you.

A WORD FROM GOD:

You have been given the privilege of trusting in Christ and also the privilege of suffering for him. Philippians 1:29

CONFESSION OF FAITH:

I will never give up fighting this cancer. Though my body is dying, my spirit is being renewed every day (see 2 Corinthians 4:16-18).

WEEK 18

Cancer Cannot Take Away My Self-Esteem

PRAYER:

How precious are Your thoughts about me, O God. They cannot be numbered! I cannot even count them. They outnumber the grains of the sand! And when I wake up, You are still with me!

(based on Psalm 139:17-18)

DEVOTIONAL:

Cancer cannot take away your self-esteem, but it will try. Chemotherapy will strip you of your hair, eyebrows and eyelashes. Burdened with fatigue, your life will become more sedentary, leading to muscle atrophy.

Chemotherapy prevents you from retaining nourishment, so you become very thin. It also makes your feet numb and painful so you cannot walk gracefully. In addition it causes short-term memory loss, which interferes with your ability to be successful in your employment. It also decreases your ability to control some body functions, and therefore you have to resort to using disposable briefs. There goes your dignity.

The world bases human worth on possessions, achievements, physical attractiveness and public acclaim. If we think like the world, then we allow cancer to take away our self-esteem. But the truth is we can feel positive about ourselves because we are made in the image of God.

> *God created human beings in his own image.*
> *In the image of God he created them;*
> *male and female he created them.*
> Genesis 1:27

> *Then God looked over all he had made, and he saw that it was very good.* Genesis 1:31

It was after God had created human beings that He declared His creation to be *"very good."*

> *Because we are united with Christ, we have received an inheritance from God, for he chose*

us in advance, and he makes everything work out according to his plan. Ephesians 1:11

When we put ourselves down we are criticizing what God has made. He sees us as being excellent in every way. When you feel worthless and of little value, remember that God made you for a reason, and cancer and chemotherapy cannot annul that plan of God. You are very valuable to Him. Your worth does not come from your achievements, but from the God of the Universe who chose to give you His free gift of life.

A WORD FROM GOD:

I knew you before I formed you in your mother's womb.
Before you were born I set you apart.
Jeremiah 1:5

CONFESSION OF FAITH:

Before God formed me in my mother's womb, He saw me and declared me to be *"very good!"*

WEEK 19

Encountering Adversity

PRAYER:

O LORD, You are a shield around me; You are my glory, the one who holds my head high. I cry out to You and You answer me. I lay down and sleep and awake in safety, for You watch over me. I am not afraid of adversity because I know that You will rescue me.

Many people say, "God will never heal her." Yet I know my victory will only come from You. Thank You for the victory, LORD God.

In Jesus' name I pray,
Amen!

DEVOTIONAL:

During your cancer journey, you will encounter tough times. Some of these times may feel like they are more than you can bear. You will wonder how you can go on. Remember that God is personally involved in your life. He has not abandoned you. Neither has He forgotten His promise of the healing that He purchased for you.

Let God use your hardship to strengthen your faith, as you continue to put your trust in Him. He is the great Burden Bearer. He is ever ready to lift you up and bear your burden. He desires that you ask for His power to help you. Nothing is too hard for the LORD (see Genesis 18:14). Let adversity drive you toward God, not away from Him.

Search for the LORD your God and listen to what He tells you (see Deuteronomy 4:29). Hold tightly without wavering to the hope that God can be trusted to keep His promises (see Hebrews 10:23).

You can always turn to God with your concerns. He is righteous in everything He does. He is filled with kindness. The LORD is close to all who call on Him in truth. He grants the desires of those who fear Him. He hears their cries for help and rescues them. The LORD protects those who love Him (see Psalm 145:17-20).

When troubles come your way, consider it an opportunity for great joy. For you know that when your faith is tested, your endurance has a chance to grow. So let it grow, for when your endurance is fully developed, you will be perfect and complete, needing nothing (see James 1:2-4).

Adversity is an opportunity for growth. You will come to know that God is with you at all times — even the rough times. He will help you and give you the strength to endure. Do not be afraid. Just have faith (see Mark 5:36).

A WORD FROM GOD:

I know about your suffering and your poverty. ... Do not be afraid of what you suffer. The devil will test you. You will suffer ... . But if you remain faithful even when facing death, I will give you the crown of life.

Revelation 2:9-10

CONFESSION OF FAITH:

I will remain faithful to the LORD my God even when facing death. When I die, He will give me the crown of life.

WEEK 20

God Is the Source of My Victory

PRAYER:

You, O Lord, live! Praise to my Rock! You deliver me from my enemies. You hold me safe beyond their reach. You save me from violent opponents. For this, O Lord, I praise You. I sing praises to Your name. You give me great victories. You have shown me Your unfailing love.

You are my King and my God. You command victories for me. Only by Your power am I able to push back the side effects of my enemy, chemotherapy. Only by Your name.

I rejoice in Your strength, O Lord! I shout for joy because You gave me the victory. You have given me my heart's desire. I asked You to preserve my life, and You granted my request. The days of my life stretch on forever.

You are the LORD of Heaven's armies. Your strong right hand is filled with victory.

(based on 2 Samuel 22:47-51,
Psalm 44:4-5, 21:1-4
and 48:8 and 10)

DEVOTIONAL:

Praise God for giving you the victory. Sing praises *to* Him, not just *about* Him. Give Him your heart. Thank Him for the victories He has promised you in His Word. Thank Him for His mercy, for His trustworthiness, for His love. Thank Him for your relationship with Him. Thank Him for your salvation and deliverance.

God will never let you down. He will stand by you and comfort you. No matter what the situation may be, the LORD is with you.

Our might is not in our weapons, but in our worship. As you worship God, you enter into His presence. It is in His presence where you will find your victory. Only God can preserve you, so place your confidence in Him.

We put our hope in the LORD.
He is our help and our shield. Psalm 33:20

A WORD FROM GOD:

Give thanks to the Lord, for he is good!
His faithful love endures forever.

1 Chronicles 16:34

CONFESSION OF FAITH:

I wait quietly before God, for my victory comes from Him (see Psalm 62:1). I will not die; instead, I will live to tell what the Lord has done (see Psalm 118:17).

WEEK 21

Declaring the Victory

PRAYER:

Your strong right arm, O LORD, has done glorious things! Your strong right arm is raised in triumph. I will not die; instead I will live to tell what You, O LORD, have done.

In Jesus' name,
Amen!

(based on Psalm 118:13-17)

DEVOTIONAL:

My enemies — cancer and chemotherapy — have done their best to kill me, but the LORD has always rescued me. The second year of this journey I suffered an intracranial hemorrhage and stroke from the chemotherapy. I came out of it with no neurological deficits.

God is my Strength and my Song. He has given me the victory. I sing songs of joy and victory in my camp (see Psalm 118:13-15).

A WORD FROM GOD:

With joy you will drink deeply
from the fountain of salvation!
In that wonderful day you will sing:
"Thank the LORD! Praise his name!
Tell the nations what he has done.
Let them know how mighty he is!
Sing to the LORD, for he has done wonderful things.
Make known his praise around the world.
Let all the people ... shout his praise with joy!
For great is the Holy One of Israel who lives among you." Isaiah 12:3-6

SONG OF PRAISE:

I thank You for answering my prayer and giving me the victory.
This is the day the LORD has made.
I will rejoice and be glad in it (see Psalm 118:24).
You are my God, and I praise You!
You are my God, and I exalt You!

I give thanks to You, O Lord, for You are good!
Your faithful love endures forever (see Psalm 118:28-29).

CONFESSION OF FAITH:

With joy I will drink deeply from the fountain of salvation!

WEEK 22

God Has Given Me the Victory

PRAYER:

O LORD my God, my enemies — chemotherapy and cancer — have done their best to kill me, but You, LORD, have rescued me. You keep me in perfect peace as I place my trust in You. You, LORD, are my eternal Rock. You have given me the victory. I thank You for Your faithfulness. I thank You for Your love. I thank You for You are trustworthy.

In Jesus' name I pray,
Amen!

DEVOTIONAL:

The cancer path is never smooth. Furthermore, it is not God's will for us. But He makes sure we are never alone as we travel it. God is there to help us, comfort us and guide us. He will give us a purpose for the journey so that we will keep our thoughts on Him. God will also make all the provisions that we need as we travel. Part of that provision is the wisdom to make decisions and the faith to trust in Him.

It is our responsibility to express our gratitude toward Him, thanking Him and praising Him and telling others about Him and what He has done for us. For we have defeated the devil by the blood of the Lamb and the word of our testimony (see Revelation 12:11).

A WORD FROM GOD:

You will keep in perfect peace
all who trust in you,
all whose thoughts are fixed on you!
Trust in the LORD always,
for the LORD GOD is the eternal Rock.

Isaiah 26:3-4

CONFESSION OF FAITH:

God has come to save me. I will trust in Him and not be afraid. The LORD God is my Strength and my Song. He has given me the victory.

WEEK 23

Wait Patiently Upon the Lord

PRAYER:

I am confident I will see Your goodness on my behalf, O LORD my God. For You are my Hiding Place. You protect me from trouble. You surround me with songs of victory.

For Your Word, O LORD, holds true, and I can trust everything You say. You are holy, enthroned in the praises of Your people.

(based on Psalm 27:13, 32:7, 33:4 and 22:3)

DEVOTIONAL:

I can stand on God's Word because it is perfectly true and absolutely trustworthy. He does not lie, forget, change His words or leave

His promises unfulfilled. I can trust His Word because it comes from a holy God (see Joshua 24:19).

God does not change. He is the same yesterday, today, and forever (see Hebrews 13:8). Since He does not change, His Word does not change. In this ever-changing world, we can always trust our unchanging LORD.

A WORD FROM GOD:

Wait patiently for the LORD.
Be brave and courageous.
Yes, wait patiently for the LORD.

Psalm 27:14

The eyes of the LORD watch over those who do right;
his ears are open to their cries for help.

Psalm 34:15

Hold firmly to the word of life.

Philippians 2:16

CONFESSION OF FAITH:

I hold firmly to the Word of Life.

WEEK 24

Waiting Quietly Before God

PRAYER:

I put my hope in You, O Lord. You are my Help and my Shield. In You, my heart rejoices, for I trust in Your holy name. Let Your unfailing love surround me, Lord. My hope is in You alone.

In Jesus' name I pray,
Amen!

(based on Psalm 33:20–22)

DEVOTIONAL:

The Lord hears His people when they call to Him for help. He rescues them from all their troubles. The Lord is close to the brokenhearted. He rescues those whose spirits are crushed. The righteous person faces many troubles, but the

LORD comes to the rescue each time. For the LORD protects the bones of the righteous, and not one of them is broken (see Psalm 34:17-20)!

As I express my feelings to God, He reaffirms my faith. When I pray, He releases the tension. As I trust Him as my Rock, my Salvation and my Fortress, my entire outlook on life changes. When I rest in God's strength, no one and nothing can shake me.

I wait quietly before God, for my victory comes from Him. He alone is my Rock and my Salvation, my Fortress. My victory and honor come from God alone. He is my Refuge, a Rock where no enemy can reach me. I trust in Him at all times. I pour out my heart to Him, for He is my Refuge (see Psalm 62:1).

A WORD FROM GOD:

Don't let your hearts be troubled. Trust in God, and also trust in me [Jesus]. John 14:1

CONFESSION OF FAITH:

I wait quietly before God, for my victory comes from Him. He alone is my Rock and my Salvation, my Fortress. My victory and honor come from God alone. He is my

Refuge, a Rock where no enemy can reach me. I trust in Him at all times. I pour out my heart to Him, for He is my Refuge.

WEEK 25

Discouragement

PRAYER:

I am so discouraged. My heart is so sad. But I will still put my hope in You, O LORD my God. I will praise You, my Savior. I am deeply discouraged, but I remember You. Each day You, O LORD, pour Your unfailing love upon me, and through each night I sing Your songs. I pray that You will give me life.

In Jesus' name,
Amen!

(based on Psalm 42:6-7)

DEVOTIONAL:

Discouragement is a common emotion associated with cancer. There are so many unanswered questions. Why me? What sin did I commit that brought this disease upon me? Why am I being punished? We tend to blame ourselves for acquiring cancer. Or we blame God.

In addition, we hope for remission. We get close, and then the tests come back positive for the return of cancer.

The cure for discouragement is focusing our thoughts on God's goodness. The LORD is our Shepherd, so we have all that we need. He lets us rest in green meadows. He leads us beside peaceful streams. He renews our strength. He guides us along right paths, bringing honor to His name.

Even when we walk through the darkest valley of death, we do not need to be afraid, for God is close beside us. His rod and His staff protect and comfort us. He prepares a feast for us in the presence of our enemies. He honors us by anointing our head with oil. Our cup overflows with blessings. His goodness and unfailing love pursues us all the days of our life, and we will live in the house of the LORD forever (see Psalm 23).

As we meditate on God's ability to help us, rather than our inability to help ourselves, the present situation loses its power over our emotional well-being. The key is to trust God and rest in His sovereignty and faithfulness.

His love endures forever. He will not fail us or abandon us.

A WORD FROM GOD:

Do not be ... discouraged, for the L*ORD* *will personally go ahead of you. ... He will neither fail you nor abandon you.*

Deuteronomy 31:8

Don't be discouraged, for I am your God.
I will strengthen you and help you.
I will hold you up with my victorious right hand. Isaiah 41:10

CONFESSION OF FAITH:

I put my hope in You, O LORD, my God.

WEEK 26

Hope in God

PRAYER:

I have put my hope in Your Word, LORD God. I thank You for promising to be with me through my rough times. Please show me how to trust You when problems arise, and give me the strength to endure them.

In Jesus' name I pray,
Amen!

(based on Psalm 119:74)

DEVOTIONAL:

You can either have your hopes or your fears fulfilled. If you reject God and follow your own desires, you will experience your fears. If you turn to God and follow Him, your hopes will be fulfilled.

God will use our life experiences to build our character and strengthen our trust in Him. So, dear brothers and sisters, when troubles come your way, consider it an opportunity for great joy. For when your faith is tested, your endurance has a chance to grow. So, let it grow, for when your endurance is fully developed, you will be perfect and complete, needing nothing (see James 1:2-4). How we react under pressure determines the depth of our character.

God will not leave you alone as you go through problems. He will stay close and help you grow. I pray that God, the source of our hope, will fill you completely with joy and peace because you trust in Him. Then you will overflow with confident hope through the power of the Holy Spirit (see Romans 15:13).

A WORD FROM GOD:

The hopes of the godly will be granted.

Proverbs 10:24

Be truly glad. There is wonderful joy ahead, even though you must endure many trials for a little while. These trials will show that your faith is genuine. It is being tested as fire tests and purifies gold — though your faith is far more precious than mere gold. So when your faith remains strong through many trials, it will bring much praise and glory and honor on the day when Jesus Christ is revealed to the world. 1 Peter 1:6-7

CONFESSION OF FAITH:

My hope is in the living God, the Savior of all people.

WEEK 27

My Hope Is in God

PRAYER:

I wait quietly before You with all that I am, LORD God, for my hope is in You. You alone are my Rock and my Salvation. My victory and honor come from You alone. You are my Refuge, a Rock where no enemy can reach me. I trust in You at all times. I pour out my heart to You, for You are my Refuge.

In Jesus' name I pray,
Amen!

(based on Psalm 62:5-8)

DEVOTIONAL:

The cancer journey is a long, dry walk down a path that will beat you up. You place your hope in the ability of chemotherapy to kill the cancer cells, and the purpose of chemotherapy is to cause the cancer cells to commit suicide and die. But they fight back and make you feel like *you* are dying. The nausea and vomiting, pain, fatigue, depression, lack of appetite, gastric distress, physical weakness, loss of memory, visual disturbances, headaches, dental pain, mouth sores, numbness in fingers and feet, forgetfulness, bloating, fluid buildup in the abdomen, etc. is all enough to make you wonder if the good cells are dying instead. And because no one understands the journey you are traveling (unless they have traveled it themselves), many have unreasonably high expectations of you. But when we rest in God's strength, nothing can shake us. Trusting God changes our entire outlook on life.

A WORD FROM GOD:

God is my strong fortress
and he makes my way perfect.

2 Samuel 22:33

CONFESSION OF FAITH:

God is my strong fortress, and He makes my way perfect.

WEEK 28

God Is Faithful to His Word

PRAYER:

O, LORD God, Your way is perfect. All Your promises prove true. You are a Shield for all who look to You for protection. You are the LORD, my solid Rock. You arm me with strength and make my way perfect. You have given me Your shield of victory. Your right hand supports me. You have made a wide path for my feet, to keep them from slipping. Thank You, my LORD.

In Jesus' name,
Amen!

(based on Psalm 18:30-36)

DEVOTIONAL:

God does not lie (see Titus 1:2). We can trust in His character because He is the truth and the source of all truth. The LORD God has given us the things He promised (see Joshua 23:15). We honor Him by believing in Him and His Word.

God is trustworthy. He keeps His promises. He bound Himself with an oath, so that those who receive the promise could be perfectly sure that He would never change His mind (see Hebrews 6:17).

We have to choose who we will believe. The choice is ours. It can be God, our own intelligence or another person. Be fully convinced that God is able to do whatever He promises (see Romans 4:21). Believe He is who He says He is. Believe He will do what He says.

Faith is the confidence that what we hope for will actually happen. It gives us assurance about things we cannot see (see Hebrews 11:1).

> *For all God's promises have been fulfilled in Christ with a resounding "Yes!" And through Christ, our "Amen" (which means "Yes") ascends to God for his glory.*
>
> 2 Corinthians 1:20

Therefore, let us hold tightly without wavering to the hope we affirm, for God can be trusted to keep His promises (see Hebrews 10:23). Remain steadfast and persevere in faith. Suffering can build our character.

Furthermore, if we let it, our suffering will help us grow in our relationship with Jesus. The Scriptures give us hope and encouragement as we wait patiently for God's promises to be fulfilled (see Romans 15:4).

A WORD FROM GOD:

I am the Lord, and I do not change.

Malachi 3:6

Patient endurance is what you need now, so that you will continue to do God's will. Then you will receive all that He has promised.

Hebrews 10:36

CONFESSION OF FAITH:

I am fully convinced that God is able to do all that He has promised.

WEEK 29

God Is My Encourager

PRAYER:

My heart is confident in you, O God;
my heart is confident.
No wonder I can sing your praises.

Psalm 57:7

DEVOTIONAL:

There will be times when we feel discouraged and abandoned by God if our healing does not come on our time, but He confesses that He is the God who heals us. He has not abandoned us and will not fail us. The Scriptures say: *"God ... encourages those who are discouraged"* (2 Corinthians 7:6), so encouragement is on the way! Let God have His perfect time.

A WORD FROM GOD:

Do not be afraid or discouraged, for the LORD will personally go ahead of you. ... He will neither fail you nor abandon you.

Deuteronomy 31:8

Be strong and courageous, and do the work. Don't be afraid or discouraged, for the LORD God ... is with you. He will not fail you or forsake you. He will see to it that all the work ... is finished correctly. 1 Chronicles 28:20

I have chosen you
and will not throw you away.
Don't be afraid, for I am with you.
Don't be discouraged, for I am your God.
I will strengthen you and help you.
I will hold you up with my victorious right hand. Isaiah 41:9-10

CONFESSION OF FAITH:

I will not be discouraged because God is holding me up with His victorious right hand.

WEEK 30

God Directs Our Steps

PRAYER:

LORD God, You direct my steps, so I will not try to understand everything along the way. I trust You fully and refuse to focus on this discouragement.

In Jesus' name I pray,
Amen!

DEVOTIONAL:

I went to a healing revival, and I knew by the physical signs I experienced that I had received healing. But when the cancer marker was drawn four days later, it was elevated. I was expecting it to be much lower. Because of this, I was so discouraged that I wept. My hopes for healing nearly diminished ... until I began writing a devotional on discouragement.

Often, the events that surround us are confusing. We try to understand them, but there will be times that we will not understand immediately ... and maybe not for years. Yet, we have to trust that God is working in the situation. That is why we never give up.

> *For our present troubles are small and won't last very long. Yet they produce for us a glory that vastly outweighs them and will last forever! So we don't look at the troubles we can see now; rather, we fix our gaze on things that cannot be seen. For the things we see now will soon be gone, but the things we cannot see will last forever.* 2 Corinthians 4:17-18

A WORD FROM GOD:

> *The LORD directs our steps,*
> *so why try to understand everything along the way?* Proverbs 20:24

CONFESSION OF FAITH:

The LORD directs my steps, so I will not try to understand everything along the way. I will maintain my trust in Him.

WEEK 31

Waiting for the Manifestation of God's Promise of Healing

PRAYER:

I waited patiently for You to help me, O Lord my God. You lifted me out of the pit of despair, out of the mud and the mire. You set my feet on solid ground and steadied me as we walked along. You have given me a new song to sing. Many will see what You have done and be amazed. They will put their trust in You, O Lord.

I have not kept the good news of Your interventions in my life hidden in my heart. I have not been afraid, as You, O Lord, well know. I have talked about Your faithfulness and saving power. I have told everyone of Your unfailing love and faithfulness.

(based on Psalm 40:1–3 and 9–10)

DEVOTIONAL:

Waiting to experience God's healing in me has not always been easy. I have gone through periods of depression. I have wondered what people were thinking. Did they think I was crazy? After all, I had told many people that God had healed me as promised in His Word. I firmly stood on this confession of my Lord's faithfulness.

Unbelievers give me reasons why I have to believe that cancer is a chronic, life-long condition, and I will eventually die from it. But I refuse to receive the reports that go against what God has promised me.

I've had periods when I wondered if I was making God look bad because the diagnosis of cancer has kept returning each time I go into remission. The whole process could have easily become a cause for me to change my confession and protect my own reputation. But I want God to get all the glory. It is all about Him, not about me.

Healing is a process that progressively takes place over time. A miracle is an instantaneous incident that surpasses human knowledge. When the Holy Spirit explained this to me, I adopted a whole new perspective on the disease and God's ability to heal it.

One day the assistant pastor of my church spoke over me, saying, "Carol, you will be fine. You will not die." Right after he spoke these words, a great burden lifted off my body, and I felt complete and whole. I had received a touch from God.

I knew that I could trust God to heal me, and I could see my healing coming. I just needed to be patient because God is not on my timetable.

> *The LORD always keeps his promises;*
> *he is gracious in all he does.* Psalm 145:13

> *He keeps every promise forever.*
> Psalm 146:6

A WORD FROM GOD:

> *The LORD isn't really being slow about his promise, as some people think. No, he is being patient for your sake.* 2 Peter 3:9

> *The LORD is my strength and my song;*
> *he has given me victory.* Exodus 15:2

But those who trust in the LORD will find new strength.
They will soar high on wings like eagles.
They will run and not grow weary.
They will walk and not faint.

Isaiah 40:31

CONFESSION OF FAITH:

The LORD is my Strength and my Song. He has given me victory.

WEEK 32

Continually Trust in the Lord

PRAYER:

O LORD, I give my life to You. I trust in You, my God! Do not let me be disgraced or let my enemies rejoice in my defeat. No one who trusts in You will ever be disgraced.

Show me the right path, O LORD. Point out the road for me to follow. Lead me by Your truth and teach me, for You are the God who saves me. All day long I put my hope in You. Remember, O LORD, Your compassion and unfailing love.

In Jesus' name I pray,
Amen!

(based on Psalm 25:1-6)

DEVOTIONAL:

King David was a man after God's own heart, and yet he faced many problems. He was scoffed at, mocked, insulted, humiliated and made the object of gossip. But he did not turn his back on God and give up.

It would be easy to turn away from God and quit trusting Him when you feel completely beaten down. It would be easy to give up this fight and give up on your commitment to serving Christ. However, it is your weakness that allows the resurrection power of Christ to strengthen you throughout the day.

There is a purpose to our suffering. Even though the situation you are going through seems hopeless, be determined to continue to pray. God hears your prayer, and He will rescue you.

A WORD FROM GOD:

Never give up. Though our bodies are dying, our spirits are being renewed every day. For our present troubles are small and won't last very long. Yet they produce for us a glory that vastly outweighs them and will last forever! So we don't look at the troubles we can see now; rather, we fix our gaze on things that cannot be seen. For the things we see now will soon be gone, but the things we cannot see will last forever. 2 Corinthians 4:16-18

CONFESSION OF FAITH:

There is life after death. I will live forever with God in a place where there is no suffering. Knowing this helps me live above my current condition.

WEEK 33

Great Is Your Faithfulness

PRAYER:

If my enemies — cancer or chemotherapy — succeed in taking my life, O Lord, many will think living for You is futile. I know my faith is intact. I know You have already won the battle. But if chemotherapy and cancer succeed, it will be an obstacle to the faith of others.

I have shared my faith and testimony with many, O Lord. You know that very well. I have watched people's faith grow. I have seen people become hungry for You and find You. People have grown in their own relationship with You. Please do not fail me or the others.

In Jesus' name I pray,
Amen!

DEVOTIONAL:

The thought of my suffering ... is bitter beyond words.
I will never forget this awful time,
as I grieve my loss.
Yet, I still dare to hope
when I remember this:
The faithful love of the LORD never ends!
His mercies never cease.
Great is his faithfulness;
his mercies begin afresh each morning.

Lamentations 3:19-23

A WORD FROM GOD:

The LORD is my inheritance;
therefore, I will hope in him!
The LORD is good to those who depend on him,
to those who search for him.
So it is good to wait quietly
for salvation from the LORD.

Laminations 3:24-26

CONFESSION OF FAITH:

No matter how desperate my situation becomes, I always know that I can call out to Jesus in faith, and He will help me.

WEEK 34

Cancer Returns

PRAYER:

All night long I pray, but my soul is not comforted. I think of You, Lord God, and I moan, overwhelmed with longing for Your help. I think of the good old days, long since ended, when my nights were filled with joyful songs. I search my soul and ponder on the difference now.

I know You have not rejected me. I know Your kindness and unfailing love endures forever. Your promises never fail. You never forget to be gracious. And You never slam the door on Your compassion.

I recall all You have done, O Lord. Your deeds are constantly in my thoughts. I cannot stop thinking about Your mighty works. Please lift me out of this discouragement, O Lord.

In Jesus' name I pray,
Amen!

(based on Psalm 77:2–11)

DEVOTIONAL:

For the fourth time — the fourth consecutive year — I have been told the cancer has returned. I feel hopeless. A year ago my faith was very strong that I was healed. I just knew that I had experienced its manifestation in my body. Remission came again in August. Now, another March has arrived, with another diagnosis of metastatic cancer.

A WORD FROM GOD:

I pray that God, the source of hope, will fill you completely with joy and peace because you trust in him. Then you will overflow with confident hope through the power of the Holy Spirit.

Romans 15:13

CONFESSION OF FAITH:

The Scriptures give me hope and encouragement, as I wait patiently for God's promises to be fulfilled (see Romans 15:4).

WEEK 35

The True Source of My Hope

PRAYER:

LORD God, it is You who brings healing to me. Forgive me for giving the glory to the chemotherapy. Yes, You use the chemo to facilitate healing, but ultimately You willingly allowed Your body to be broken so that You could purchase the healing for my broken body. So, despite all the side effects from the chemotherapy, You give me life. And I give You all the glory.

In Jesus' name I pray,
Amen!

DEVOTIONAL:

Since I placed my hope in the ability of chemotherapy to get me into remission and healed, I struggle to hang on to my faith that God will fulfill His promise of healing in my body, now that I have received the fourth diagnosis of metastatic cancer. I had expected the drug to cause all those cancer cells to commit suicide and never return.

A WORD FROM GOD:

I am the Lord who heals you.

Exodus 15:26

By his wounds
you are healed. 1 Peter 2:24

It was our weaknesses he carried;
it was our sorrows that weighed him down.
And we thought his troubles were a punishment from God,
a punishment for his own sins!
But he was pierced for our rebellion,
crushed for our sins.
He was beaten so we could be whole.
He was whipped so we could be healed.

Isaiah 53:4-5

He himself gives life and breath to everything,
and he satisfies every need.

His purpose was for the nations to seek after God and perhaps feel their way toward him and find him — though he is not far from any one of us. For in him we live and move and exist. Acts 17:25 and 27-28

CONFESSION OF FAITH:

In God I live, and move and exist.

WEEK 36

God Is My Savior

PRAYER:

I love You, Lord. You are my Strength. You are my Rock, my Fortress and my Savior. You are God, my Rock, in whom I find protection. You are my Shield, the power that saves me from my enemies. The ropes of death entangled me. The grave wrapped its ropes around me. Death laid a trap in my path. But in my distress I cried out to You. Yes, I prayed to You for help.

You heard me from Your sanctuary. My cry reached Your ears. You reached down from Heaven and rescued me. You rescued me from my powerful enemies — cancer and chemotherapy — who were too strong for me. You supported me. You led me to a place of safety.

You rescued me because You delighted in me. You rewarded me for doing right. You have seen my innocence. To the faithful, You show Yourself faithful. To those with integrity, You show integrity. To the pure, You show Yourself pure. But to the wicked, You show Yourself hostile.

You rescue the humble, but You humiliate the proud. You light a lamp for me. You, O LORD my God, light up my darkness. By Your strength You crushed my enemies.

Your way is perfect. All of Your promises prove true. You are a shield for all who look to You for protection. You arm me with strength, and make my way perfect. You have given me Your shield of victory. Your right hand supports me.

Amen!

(based on Psalm 18:1-6, 16-32 and 35)

DEVOTIONAL:

There is no limit to God's protection. It can take many forms. He is the Most High God. When I was defenseless, God moved in and rescued me from my enemies — cancer and chemotherapy.

I have been fighting the good fight for four years. The first year I had cancer I went through a deep grieving process. I came out of my first year of chemotherapy with a more intimate relationship with God and a deeper faith.

The second year with cancer I developed an intracranial hemorrhage from the chemotherapy and had a stroke. The neurological deficits from that stroke have resolved.

The third year of chemotherapy, it was expected that my heart would be enlarged after the course of treatment and be weaker. But my heart was stronger after I had finished this course chemotherapy than it had been before I started it.

The fourth year of cancer I was supposed to lose my quality of life and be admitted to Hospice. I have yet to experience either of these circumstances. However, I have now been given four months to live. I excitedly await God's intervention in this report. I fully expect Him to glorify Himself.

As I look back on the journey that I have traveled, battling the cancer and side effects from chemotherapy, I am amazed at how far my Lord God has brought me. How could I doubt His ability to heal me? My relationship with Him has become so intimately personal. My faith and trust in Him is so strong. I am thankful for this opportunity to come into a deeper knowledge of Him, even though I had to suffer to acquire it.

Sometimes God does not rescue us from our troubles immediately. Instead, He becomes our support as we go through them. He claims it as His time to reveal Himself to us in a new way so that we can know Him more intimately.

A WORD FROM GOD:

Call on me when you are in trouble and I will rescue you, and you will give me the glory.

Psalm 50:15

CONFESSION OF FAITH:

You are my Strength, O LORD. You are my Rock, my Fortress and my Savior, in whom I find protection. You are my Shield, the power that saves me, and my place of safety.

SONG OF PRAISE:

My LORD lives!
All praise to my Rock!
Let the God of my Salvation be exalted!
You rescued me from my enemies.
For this, O LORD, I sing praises to Your name.
You have given me a great victory!
You have showered me with Your unfailing love!

WEEK 37

Our Sovereign Lord

PRAYER:

O Sovereign Lord, You have only begun to show Your greatness and the strength of Your hand to me, Your servant. You have given me four years of life, when I was given only five months. You kept me neurologically intact when I had a brain hemorrhage from chemotherapy that caused a stroke. You made my heart stronger when chemotherapy was supposed to enlarge it and make it weaker. You maintained my quality of life when I was told I would lose it in two months. You sustained me financially when it looked like I was going to start losing my possessions. You have met my every need during this troubled journey. Is there any god in Heaven or on Earth who can perform such great and mighty deeds as You do?

Please show them all Your glory, LORD, and extend my life by many years. My heart rejoices in You, O LORD! You have made me strong. Now I have an answer for my enemies. I rejoice because You have rescued me. No one is holy like You! There is no one but You. There is no rock like my God.

In Jesus' name I pray,
Amen!

(based on Deuteronomy 3:24 and 1 Samuel 2:1-2)

DEVOTIONAL:

God promises to help us win every battle we must endure so we have nothing to fear. He fights with us and for us, as we place our hope in Him. Our part of the battle consists of having confidence in God and gratitude for all that He has done and will continue to do. He is ultimately in control over the events of our lives. Be thankful for the ways He blesses you.

A WORD FROM GOD:

Continue to believe that Jesus is the Messiah, the Son of God. ... By believing in him you will have life by the power of his name.

John 20:31

CONFESSION OF FAITH:

Our Sovereign Lord is great! There is no one like Him (see 2 Samuel 7:22).

WEEK 38

Our Victory Comes from God

PRAYER:

Not to me, not to the doctors, not to the chemotherapy, but to Your name goes all the glory, my LORD, for Your unfailing love and faithfulness.

I trust only in You, O LORD! You are my Helper and my Shield. I praise You, LORD. I thank You for answering my prayer and giving me the victory!

You are my God and I praise You. You are my God and I exalt You.

In Jesus' name I pray,
Amen!

(based on Psalm 115:1 and 10 and 118:21

DEVOTIONAL:

We are blessed by the LORD who made Heaven and Earth (see Psalm 115:15). He loves us with unfailing love. His faithfulness endures forever (see Psalm 117:2). Give thanks to the LORD, for He is good! His faithful love endures forever.

My enemies — chemotherapy and cancer — have done their best to kill me, but the LORD rescued me each time. The LORD is my Strength and my Song. He has given me victory. The strong right arm of the LORD has done glorious things (see Psalm 118:1, 13-14 and 16).

God stays close to us, even when we are near death. We are precious to Him, and He carefully chooses the time when He will call us home. Our life is valuable to Him. Praise the LORD. He will comfort us. He came to save us. Trust in Him, and do not be afraid.

SONG OF PRAISE:

I praise You, O LORD!
You comfort me.
You came to save me.
I trust in You and will not be afraid.
You are my Strength and my Song.

You have given me the victory.
With joy I drink deeply from the fountain of salvation!
Thank You, LORD!
I praise Your name!
I will tell them what You have done.
I will let them know how mighty You are.
You have done wonderful things.
I will make known Your praise around the world.
I will shout Your praises with joy.
For You are great, O Holy One!

(based on Isaiah 12)

A WORD FROM GOD:

Praise the LORD!
Sing to the LORD a new song.
Sing His praises in the assembly of the faithful.
Rejoice in your Maker.
... Exult in your King.
For the LORD delights in His people;
He crowns the humble with victory. ...
Sing for joy as [you] lie on [your] bed.

Psalm 149:1-5

CONFESSION OF FAITH:

Overwhelming victory is mine through Christ Jesus (see Romans 8:37)

WEEK 39

Take Refuge in the Lord

PRAYER:

Lord God, You are with me, so I have no fear. I know You will help me. You are Sovereign, and I take refuge in You. I place my trust in You alone. Chemotherapy offers nothing in which I can place my trust.

DEVOTIONAL:

I frequently ask myself how much longer I can go on with these yearly diagnoses of metastatic cancer. I was first diagnosed in March, then went into remission in August. I was diagnosed again the following March, and then went into remission that August. The process repeated itself the following March and August. But last year I came out of remission too soon. The cancer returned, and my oncologist told me remission would not be a possibility this time. I feel so abandoned by the Word of God. My prognosis, according to my physician, is very poor. She has given me only four months to live. I am now on disability and spend much time and energy worrying about being able to meet my financial obligations and wondering how to handle the healthcare issues, should there be no medical insurance.

A WORD FROM GOD:

I will not fail you or abandon you.

Joshua 1:5

CONFESSION OF FAITH:

The Lord my God will not fail me nor abandon me.

WEEK 40

God Is Able to Restore My Life

PRAYER:

I exalt You, LORD, for You rescued me. You refused to let my enemies — chemotherapy and cancer — triumph over me. O LORD my God, I cried to You for help, and You restored my health. You brought me up from the grave, O LORD. You kept me from falling into the pit of death. I give You all the glory.

In Jesus' name,
Amen!

(based on Psalm 30:1-3)

DEVOTIONAL:

God is able to give me back my life despite what chemotherapy and cancer try to take away. This journey is only a temporary condition for me. The tears that I have shed will bring a harvest of joy, because God is able to bring good out of cancer and chemotherapy. My grief is temporary, and I will again experience joy.

A WORD FROM GOD:

Those who plant in tears
will harvest with shouts of joy.
They weep as they go to plant their seed,
but they sing as they return with harvest.

Psalm 126:5-6

CONFESSION OF FAITH:

I wait patiently for God's great harvest of joy.

WEEK 41

No More Chemotherapy

PRAYER:

I thank You for answering my prayer and giving me the victory. You are my God, and I praise You! You are my God, and I exalt You! I give thanks to You, O LORD, for You are good! Your faithful love endures forever.

In Jesus' name I pray,
Amen!

(based on Psalm 118:28–29)

DEVOTIONAL:

I have been told that the day is coming when chemotherapy is no longer going to be available to me because it will lose its value in my treatment. The oncologist has told me that I will never see remission again. Chemotherapy has been my source of hope for the last four years. As I envision that bag hanging on the intravenous pole above me, I see a plastic bag filled with fluid that has become a god in which I have placed my trust and faith for staying alive.

My enemies — cancer and chemotherapy — have done their best to kill me, but the LORD has always rescued me. He is my Strength and my Song. He has given me victory. I sing songs of joy and victory in my camp. His strong right arm has done glorious things! His strong right arm is raised in triumph. I will not die. Instead, I will live to tell what the LORD has done (see Psalm 118:13-17).

In my distress I prayed to the LORD, and the LORD answered me and set me free. The LORD is for me, so I will have no fear. What can cancer do to me? Yes, the LORD is for me. He will help me. It is better to take refuge in the LORD than to trust in chemotherapy (see Psalm 118:5-8).

A WORD FROM GOD:

> *You must not bow down to it and worship it, for I, the LORD your God am a jealous God who will not tolerate your affection for any other gods.* Exodus 20:5

If we confess our sins to him, he is faithful and just to forgive us our sins and to cleanse us from all wickedness. 1 John 1:9

CONFESSION OF SIN:

O Lord God, forgive me for allowing chemotherapy to become the god that gives me life. Thank You for Your faithfulness to forgive me of this sin and cleanse me from the wickedness of making chemotherapy the god of my life. Lord God, You are for me, so I have no fear as to what cancer can do to me. I know You will help me. You are sovereign, and I take refuge in You. I place my trust in You alone, for chemotherapy offers nothing in which I can place my trust. Chemotherapy has proven itself untrustworthy. I denounce it as a god in my life.

Amen!

CONFESSION OF FAITH:

The Lord has set me free. The Lord is for me, so I will have no fear. He will help me. I take refuge in the Lord and place my trust in Him alone.

WEEK 42

It Is Finished

PRAYER:

I praise You, O Lord. With my whole heart I praise You. I praise Your holy name. With all that I am I praise You. I will never forget all the good things that You have done for me. You have forgiven all my sins. You have healed all my diseases. You have redeemed me from death. You have crowned me with Your everlasting love and tender mercies. You have filled my life with good things. You have renewed my youth. I praise You O Lord.

In Jesus' name I pray,
Amen!

(based on Psalm 103:1-5)

DEVOTIONAL:

As Jesus hung on the cross, the Scriptures show:

Jesus knew that his mission was now finished, and to fulfill Scripture he said, "I am thirsty." A jar of sour wine was sitting there, so they soaked a sponge in it, put it on a hyssop branch, and held it up to his lips. When Jesus had tasted it, he said, "It is finished!" Then he bowed his head and released his spirit.

John 19:28-30

Jesus had fought the pain of the wounds He had to bear and the nails in His hands and feet. He had hung on the cross naked in the sun for hours. He had lost a massive amount of blood from His wounds due to the torture He had endured. He was very thirsty. The soldiers offered Him sour wine to drink. He felt abandoned by the Father — left for dead. Yet He also knew the beginning from the end of His ministry. And this was just the beginning of the fantastic end that was coming!

In like manner, we have suffered under the influence of chemotherapy and cancer. We have suffered through the side effects and also from the cancer itself. We have questioned God, "What is the use of all this suffering?" But, like Jesus, we can be sure that the end of our journey will be better than the beginning.

A WORD FROM GOD:

Keep a clear mind in every situation. Don't be afraid of suffering for the Lord. Work at telling others the Good News, and fully carry out the ministry God has set before you.

2 Timothy 4:5

CONFESSION OF FAITH:

I am not afraid of suffering for the LORD because it gives me the opportunity to tell others of the Good News and fully carry out the ministry God has set before me.

WEEK 43

I Will Not Suffer

PRAYER:

O LORD, my God, You made the whole world and everything in it. Since You are LORD of Heaven and Earth, You do not live in man-made temples, and human hands cannot serve Your needs (for You have no needs). You Yourself give life and breath to everything, and You satisfy every need.

Your purpose was for the nations to seek after You and perhaps feel their way toward You and find You — though You are not far from any one of us. For in You we live, and move and exist.

You are alive, and I do not think of You as an idol designed by craftsmen from gold or silver or stone. You are the one true God. You alone are worthy of all my praise and worship.

In Jesus' name I pray,
Amen!

(based on Acts 17:24–28)

DEVOTIONAL:

God promised that if we will listen carefully to the voice of the LORD our God and do what is right in His sight, obeying His commands and keeping all His decrees, then He would not make us suffer any of the diseases that He sent upon the Egyptians, for, he said, *"I am the LORD [Jehovah Rapha] who heals you"* (Exodus 15:26).

This word *heal* means "to mend [become better in a health sense]; to cure [return to a healthy condition]; to make whole [regain sound health]; and to restore to health [bring back to health and vigor]." Since the LORD God is the source of my healing, He is ultimately the one who mends me, cures me, makes me whole and restores me to health.

The LORD promised that if the Israelites obeyed Him, they would not suffer from the diseases that plagued the Egyptians. This promise is for me also. A promise is a ground for hope and expectation — a covenant between me and the LORD. He did not say I would not get sick. He said I would not *"suffer"* from the disease ... if I obey. In other words, I would not feel unbearable pain or distress. I would not experience the extreme complications of the disease. I would be able to endure whatever comes my way.

This has certainly been true during my personal four-year journey. When my father developed metastatic lung cancer, he was very sick from the chemotherapy and radiation. He vomited continually. He had extreme pain wherever the radiation hit his body. He turned orange after going into liver failure and lost so much weight that he was unrecognizable. At the same time, he experienced hallucinations, as he withdrew from alcoholism, eventually going into a coma and dying.

I did not receive radiation, but I went into chemotherapy expecting the worst. I was not ready to face all the nausea and vomiting. I do not like to vomit. However, the nausea and vomiting was very limited and bearable due to the medications I received before the administration of the chemotherapy. In addition, I was prescribed medications to take for three days after chemotherapy that also prevented nausea and vomiting. This was such a blessing for me. That was one fear I did not have to face.

There is a spirit within people, the breath of the Almighty within them, that makes them intelligent (see Job 32:8). I praise God for giving wisdom to those in the medical field regarding these medications.

The worst part of chemotherapy for me was the severe fatigue and the memory loss. Eventually, the neuropathy threatened my ability to function. I had always been very active, and I felt I had to keep working so as not to lose my health insurance benefits. As a single person, I had to take my financial situation into consideration. So I continued to work despite my inability to fully function. During that time, I drew upon the strength of my LORD and pushed through.

God promises blessings to be fulfilled based upon an act of obedience. *"If you will listen carefully to the voice of the LORD your God and do what is right in his sight, obeying his commands and keeping all his decrees ..."* The LORD designed many of the moral laws in His Word to keep us free from sickness and harm. If I want God to care for me, then I must submit to His directions for living my daily life.

God, the LORD, created the heavens and stretched them out.
He created the earth and everything in it.

He gives breath to everyone,
life to everyone who walks on the earth.

Isaiah 42:5

For the Spirit of God has made me,
and the breath of the Almighty gives me life.

Job 33:4

A WORD FROM GOD:

I carried you on eagles' wings, and brought you to myself. Now if you will obey me and keep my covenant, you will be my own special treasure from among all the peoples on earth, for the earth belongs to me. Exodus 19:4-5

CONFESSION OF FAITH:

The Lord my God is never far from me, for in Him I live and move and exist. He gives life and breath to me and satisfies my every need.

WEEK 44

My Comfort Comes from God

PRAYER:

LORD God, I may be pressed on every side by troubles, but I am not crushed. I may be perplexed, but I am not driven to despair. I may be hunted down, but I am never abandoned by You. I get knocked down, but I am not destroyed.

Through suffering, my body continues to share in the death of Jesus, so that the life of Jesus may also be seen in my body. O LORD my God, throughout this cancer journey, You have carried me on eagles' wings and brought me to Yourself. Thank You for never leaving or forsaking me.

In Jesus' name I pray,
Amen!

(based on 2 Corinthians 4:8–10)

DEVOTIONAL:

Though I may think that I am at the end of my rope, I am never at the end of my hope. My perishable body is subject to suffering, but God has never abandoned me. I have eternal life because Christ won the victory over death. All my suffering is an opportunity for Christ to demonstrate His power and presence in and through me.

I look to God for my strength. When suffering threatens to rob me of the victory, I remind myself that nothing can destroy what God has accomplished through me.

I never give up. Though my body is dying, my spirit is being renewed every day. For my present troubles are small and will not last very long. Yet they produce for me a glory that vastly outweighs them and will last forever! So I do not look at the troubles I can see now. Rather, I fix my gaze on things that cannot be seen. For the things I see now will soon be gone, but the things I cannot see will last forever (see 2 Corinthians 4:11-18).

I know that one day I will obtain God's rest and reward. As I face my own suffering, it would be easy to focus upon the pain rather than the ultimate goal. Just as an athlete focuses on the finish line and ignores the discomfort, I, too, must focus upon the reward for my faith and the joy that lasts forever. No matter what happens to me in this life, I have the assurance of eternal life, when all this suffering will end, and all the sorrow will flee away.

It would be easy to lose heart and quit. I have frequently thought about giving up. Instead, I concentrate on the inner strength that comes from the Holy Spirit. My weakness allows the resurrection power of Christ to strengthen me moment by moment. As I journey through this terrible illness, with its pain, it reminds me that this life is not all there is. There is life after death. I will live forever with God in a place without sin and suffering. This helps me live above the pain that I experience in this life.

God has prepared a way for me to travel to His home. He does not simply point me in the right direction; He walks beside me.

All praise to God, the Father of my LORD Jesus Christ. God is my merciful Father and the source of all comfort. He comforts me in all my troubles so that I can comfort others. When they are troubled, I will be able to give them the same comfort God has given me. For the more I suffer for Christ, the more God will shower me with His comfort through Christ. So, even when I am weighed down with troubles, it is for your comfort and salvation! For when I myself am comforted, I will certainly comfort you. Then you can patiently endure the same things I suffer. I am confident that as you share in my sufferings, you will also share in the comfort God gives me (see 2 Corinthians 1:3-7).

When God comforts me, my troubles do not necessarily go away. If that were the case, people would not turn to God out of love, but, instead, out of a need to be relieved of pain. Being comforted means receiving strength, encouragement and hope to deal with my troubles. The more I suffer the more God comforts me. Every trial that I endure on this journey is for the purpose of comforting others who are on the same journey. I suffer for the Gospel, just as Jesus suffered for it. I rejoice in my suffering because I am drawing people closer to Christ. In addition, my faith has grown, and my relationship with God has deepened in a way I never thought imaginable. God has used my suffering to make me a better Christian.

A WORD FROM GOD:

The LORD watches over those who fear him,
those who rely upon his unfailing love.
He rescues them from death
and keeps them alive in times of famine.

Psalm 33:18-19

CONFESSION OF FAITH:

I may be pressed on every side by troubles, but I am not crushed. I may be perplexed, but I am not driven to despair. I may be hunted down, but I am never abandoned by God. I might get knocked down, but I am not destroyed. Through suffering, my body shares in the death of Jesus, so that the life of Jesus may be seen in my body.

WEEK 45

Bring All Your Troubles to God

PRAYER:

I praise You, LORD. I praise You, God, my Savior, for each day You carry me in Your arms. You, O God, are a God who saves! You, O Sovereign LORD, rescue me from death. I rely on Your caring strength, LORD God.

In Jesus' name,
Amen!

(based on Psalm 68:19-20)

DEVOTIONAL:

I do not have to carry all my troubles as I travel this cancer journey. God wants me to give them to Him. He wants to remove my burden from my shoulders. He wants to bear the report that the cancer may have metastasized to my brain. He wants to take the cough and sore throat and the associated temperature of 101°. He wants to bear the weight loss. He even wants to handle the flat tire. All the troubles I encounter on this journey make me weary, yet nothing is too big for God. And nothing is too small or too insignificant for Him either. If it concerns me, it concerns Him. The Scriptures tell me to turn my worries into prayers.

> *Do not worry about anything; instead pray about everything. Tell God what you need, and thank him for all He has done. Then you will experience God's peace, which exceeds anything we can understand. His peace will guard your hearts and minds as you live in Christ Jesus.*
>
> Philippians 4:6-7

The Scriptures also tell me that God so deeply cares about me that He has numbered the very hairs on my head:

> *The very hairs on your head are all numbered. So do not be afraid; you are more valuable to God than a whole flock of sparrows.*
>
> Luke 12:7

God cares for me because I belong to Him. I am very valuable to Him. He did not put me on this journey, but He carries me as I travel it.

A WORD FROM GOD:

I will rescue those who love me.
I will protect those who trust in my name.
When they call on me, I will answer;
I will be with them in trouble.
I will rescue and honor them.
I will reward them with a long life
and give them my salvation.

Psalm 91:14-16

CONFESSION OF FAITH:

God, my Savior, carries me in His arms as I travel this journey each day.

WEEK 46

God Fights My Battles

PRAYER:

O Lord my God, You are going ahead of me. You will fight for me. I will not be afraid. I will not be discouraged by the chemotherapy and cancer. The battle is not mine, but Yours, O God.

In Jesus' name I pray,
Amen!

(based on Deuteronomy 1:30 and 2 Chronicles 20:15)

DEVOTIONAL:

God has promised to fight with me and for me, as I place my hope and confidence in Him during this journey. I could complain about my situation, but it would only breed negativity, which leads to fear and immobility. God has given me His promises to focus on. As I meditate on His Word, I learn to trust Him and to overcome the negatives. My problems cannot rob me of my victory. Nevertheless I do not rely upon my own strength during the battle. I ask God for His help when I face struggles. I know God will fight for me, and He always wins. So I stand still and watch, as the Lord rescues me.

A WORD FROM GOD:

Do not be afraid … for the Lord your God will fight for you. Deuteronomy 3:22

CONFESSION OF FAITH:

I may be up against a strong enemy, but I have the Lord my God to help me and to fight the battle for me (see 2 Chronicles 32:8).

WEEK 47

Why Me?

PRAYER:

O Lord, You are a God of compassion and mercy, filled with unfailing love and faithfulness. Look down and have mercy on me. Give Your strength to Your servant, and save me.

In Jesus' name I pray,
Amen!

(based on Psalm 86:15-16)

DEVOTIONAL:

The suffering I have been enduring has become increasingly intense. I am losing weight rapidly and have become very thin. This is a grave concern for my oncologist. As I increase my portion size at mealtime, I become nauseated, vomiting at times. Eating has become a fearful experience, so I lose more weight.

Now my mouth is filled with painful ulcers from the chemotherapy, and eating only increases the pain and the size of the ulcers. So I eat my meals through a straw. I feel so defeated in my attempt to gain weight. I am reminded of Job.

Job was a wealthy man with an abundance of possessions and a large family. He was also a great judge who was admired by everyone for his wisdom. He was very content, for he had everything he could ever want. Furthermore, Job loved God and lived a blameless life before Him.

Then one day Satan came before God and asked for permission to destroy Job. God granted him that permission ... as long as he did not take Job's life. Satan immediately destroyed Job's flocks, all his possessions, his children and his health. All Job had left was his wife and a body covered with painful boils.

Job was in so much pain that he cursed the day he was born, but he did not give up on God — even though he did not understand why all of this had happened to him. Instead, he continued to trust God, no matter what happened. He was encouraged by his wife to curse God, blaming Him for all their suffering, but Job refused.

Although God loves us, believing and obeying Him does not protect us from life's tragedies, sorrows and sufferings. But, if we let them, these adversities will cause us to dig our roots deeper into God. He is fully aware of every attempt by Satan to bring suffering and calamity upon us. Satan uses these strategies to draw us away from God. Although God may allow us to suffer for reasons beyond our understanding, He is still moved with compassion for us in our suffering.

A WORD FROM GOD:

For the Lord has comforted his people
and will have compassion on them in their suffering. Isaiah 49:13

CONFESSION OF FAITH:

God will comfort me and have compassion on me in my sufferings.

WEEK 48

If Death Draws Near

PRAYER:

O Lord, when I die, You will not leave my soul among the dead or allow me to rot in the grave. You will show me the way of life, granting me the joy of Your presence and the pleasures of living with You forever.

(based on Psalm 16:10)

DEVOTIONAL:

Yesterday my oncologist gave me four months to live. If I stay on the chemotherapy, then I have four months before the side effects take my life. If I stop the chemotherapy, then I have four months before the cancer takes it. This news has cast an emotional dark shadow over me. I fear the unknown. What is the end going to be like for me? I pray that it is peaceful.

Death does not have the final word for me. First of all, man does not call me home; God calls me home. When I do walk through that dark valley of death, I will not be afraid for the LORD my God remains close beside me (see Psalm 23:4). The LORD is my Light and Salvation, so why should I be afraid? The Lord is my Fortress, protecting me from danger, so why should I tremble (see Psalm 27:1)? God will walk me through that dark valley and bring me safely to the other side. He will not forget me when I die. He will bring me to life again, to live with Him forever. Death is not a dark door at the end of my life. It is a bright pathway to a new and better life.

The LORD cares deeply when His loved ones die (see Psalm 49:10). He will stay close to me in death. I am precious to Him and He carefully chooses the time that He will call me into His presence.

A WORD FROM GOD:

The way of the godly leads to life; that path does not lead to death. Proverbs 12:28

CONFESSION OF FAITH:

When I walk through the dark valley of death, I will not be afraid, for the Lord my God remains close beside me.

WEEK 49

All to the Glory of God

PRAYER:

Not to me, O LORD, not to me, but to Your name goes all the glory. I trust You for You are my Helper and my Shield.

(based on Psalm 115:1 and 9)

DEVOTIONAL:

Nothing is impossible with God. Doing the impossible is everyday business for Him. He can take the death sentence spoken over me and turn it into an opportunity for His glory.

The situation will try to paralyze me because it seems humanly impossible to escape it, but concentrating on God and His power will help me see the way out. So I will focus on God and trust Him for the way out because He can open up a way and deliver on what He promises.

He always delivers on time, meaning at the proper time. So I will maintain an attitude of expectancy.

> *Faith is the confidence that what we hope for will actually happen; it gives us assurance about things we cannot see.* Hebrews 11:1

A WORD FROM GOD:

> *I have refined you, but not as silver is refined. Rather, I have refined you in the furnace of suffering.* Isaiah 48:10

CONFESSION OF FAITH:

> *The word of God will never fail.*
> Luke 1:37

WEEK 50

Enter the Rest

PRAYER:

When doubts try to fill my mind, Your comfort, O Lord, gives me renewed hope and cheer. My heart is confident in You. I sing Your praises.

(based on Psalm 57:7 and 94:19)

DEVOTIONAL:

In May of 2011, I had my first dose of chemotherapy. Now I am told that in May of 2015 I will die either from the chemotherapy or the cancer. I ask God, "How can this be? I have patiently waited for the manifestation of Your healing in my body. Your Word says that I am healed by Christ's wounds (see 1 Peter 2:24).

This word *healed* is past tense. It is already a done deal. I can see it. I feel I can reach out and touch it. Doubts try to fill my mind, but because of my faith in Jesus Christ, my heart and mind are filled with the peace of God that exceeds anything I can understand.

I rest in that peace. That is where God wants me right now. He wants me to enter that "*rest*":

> *We who believe can enter his rest.*
>
> Hebrews 4:3

It is in that rest that I expectantly await the manifestation of my healing — to the glory of God.

> *For a peaceful heart leads to a healthy body.*
>
> Proverbs 14:30

A WORD FROM GOD:

> *Don't let your hearts be troubled. Trust in God, and trust also in me [Jesus].* John 14:1

> *Don't be afraid, for I am with you.*
> *Don't be discouraged, for I am your God.*
> *I will strengthen you and help you.*
> *I will hold you up with my victorious right hand.* Isaiah 41:10

Do not be afraid, for I have ransomed you.
I have called you by name; you are mine.

Isaiah 43:1

CONFESSION OF FAITH:

By His wounds I am healed.

WEEK 51

There Is Healing in Communion

DEVOTIONAL:

In the church, our pastors lead us through Holy Communion in an orderly manner. However, outside of the church, if you are a Christian, you are part of a royal priest. The Scriptures say:

> *You are a chosen people. You are royal priests, a holy nation, God's very own possession. As a result, you can show others the goodness of God, for he called you out of the darkness into his wonderful light.* 1 Peter 2:9

This qualifies you to partake of the LORD's table at home — by yourself or with others.

If you are sick, partake of the LORD's supper often, and release your faith for His forgiveness and healing. There is no limitation on how often we can partake of Holy Communion.

> *For every time you eat this bread and drink this cup, you are proclaiming the Lord's death until he comes again.* 1 Corinthians 11:26

So, as often as you partake, you partake of Jesus' health and wholeness.

See the Communion as medicine. Doctors prescribe medicine to be taken daily, sometimes twice a day, three times a day or even four times a day. How often you partake of the heavenly medicine is between you and God, our Great Physician —Jehovah Rapha —the LORD who heals you.

Before partaking, prayerfully ask the Father what you want this *"cup of blessing"* to do in your life.

PRAYER:

Father, You are my Healer — Jehovah Rapha — the God who heals me. I boldly come before Your throne and ask that You heal me of cancer. The Scriptures say:

> *Yet it was our weaknesses he carried;*
> *it was our sorrows that weighed him down.*

And we thought his troubles were a punishment from God,
a punishment for his own sins!
But he was pierced for our rebellion,
crushed for our sins.
He was beaten so we could be whole.
He was whipped so we could be healed.

Isaiah 53:4-5

I boldly come before You and receive my healing by faith.

In Jesus' name I pray,
Amen!

Now, taking the Communion elements in your hand, give thanks for them.

Thank You, Jesus, for the sacrament of Communion.

Hear Jesus saying to you:

I am the bread of life! Your ancestors ate the manna in the wilderness, but they all died. Anyone who eats the bread from heaven, however, will never die. I am the living bread

> *from heaven. Anyone who eats this bread will live forever, and this bread, which I will offer so the world may live, is my flesh.*
>
> John 6:48-51

Remember: *"It was our weaknesses he carried, it was our sorrows that weighed him down"* (Isaiah 53:4). See Jesus carrying all your sins and diseases. He took your sins in His body on the cross, and He took your physical condition on His body as well. See your physical condition on His body. It is no longer on you, so you no longer have to carry it.

Release your faith in the bread and the wine. Hold the bread in your hand and pray:

PRAYER:

I give thanks to You, Jesus, for Your broken body. You willingly allowed Your body to be broken so that You could purchase my healing. I thank You that by Your stripes, by the beatings You bore, by the lashes that fell on Your back, I am completely healed. I believe, and I receive.

Hear Jesus saying to you:

> *This is my body, which is broken for you. Do this to remember me.* 1 Corinthians 11:24.

Anyone who eats my flesh and drinks my blood abides in me, and I in him. John 6:56

Eat the bread, and see His health come upon you as He abides in you.

Now take the cup in your hand and pray:

PRAYER:

Thank You, Jesus, for the new covenant cut in Your blood. Your shed blood has purchased my forgiveness and washed me from every sin. I give thanks to You because Your blood has made me righteous. As I drink, I celebrate and partake of the inheritance of the righteous, which is preservation, healing, wholeness and prosperity.

See Jesus' eyes burning with love for you, as He says:

This cup is the new covenant between God and his people — an agreement confirmed with my blood for you. Do this to remember me as often as you drink it. 1 Corinthians 11:25

Now drink the cup, laying hold of all the benefits of Jesus Christ's full redemption for your life — forgiveness, wholeness, strength, health and, sufficiency — all through this *"cup of blessing."* See Jesus carrying all your sins and diseases. He took them in His body on the cross. See them on His body. They are no longer on you.

Now pray this:

PRAYER:

I thank You, Jesus. I love You because You first loved me.

Communion is an exchange, and an *exchange* is "the laying aside of a thing, state, or condition and taking another in its place." Jesus came to exchange our unrighteousness for His righteousness, our penalty of death for His promise of life everlasting, our weakness for His strength, our sickness for His healing and our chastisement for His peace. When we understand the power and place of the LORD's supper in our lives, we will walk in divine health. It is the birthright of our covenant relationship with God.

Each time you approach the LORD's table, actively call to mind His death. Partaking of the bread and wine is not a ritual. It is an act of worship. Take hold of all that Jesus purchased for you through His cross now.

CONFESSION OF FAITH:

I am healed!

WEEK 52

God Holds My Future in His Hands

PRAYER:

Teach me Your ways, O LORD, that I may live according to Your truth! Grant me purity of heart, so that I may honor You. With all my heart I will praise You, O LORD my God. I will give glory to Your name forever, for Your love for me is very great. You have rescued me from the depths of death.

(based on Psalm 86:11–13)

DEVOTIONAL:

Not everything that happens to me is good. Cancer is not good. But God *is* good, and He is able to turn the cancer around for my good. He always works toward His purpose for me.

I knew you before I formed you in your mother's womb. Before you were born I set you apart and appointed you for a purpose. Jeremiah 1:5

Before I was even a glimmer in my mother's eye, God knew that I was going to suffer with cancer at this time in my life. That did not stop Him from appointing me to the work He wanted to accomplish through me for His glory. He decided then that cancer would not interfere with that work. Instead He would use cancer to complete the work.

"I know the plans I have for you," says the LORD. *"They are plans for good and not for disaster, to give you a future and a hope."*
Jeremiah 29:11

God knows my future. He holds it in His hands. He believes that I can do the task He has set before me, and He will be with me the whole journey. So I move forward, full of hope that God will see me through to a glorious conclusion.

God is full of surprises. If I focus only on what the doctor has said about my future, then I will only see a road that has a dead end. But that road block is merely an illusion. My future is in

God's hands, and He can do surprising things with it.

God surprised me just today. Every month I have what is called a CA (carbohydrate antigen) 125 drawn. It is a cancer indicator that tells the oncologist if the cancer is growing and spreading. The indicator had dropped by 524 points and is now down to 367.8, which is the lowest it has been for more than a year. I feel great physically, and I give God all the glory. *I Still Live.*

A WORD FROM GOD:

For I am about to do something new.
See, I have already begun! Do you not see it?
I will make a pathway through the wilderness.
I will create rivers in the dry wasteland.

Isaiah 43:19

CONFESSION OF FAITH:

God holds my future in His hands, and *I STILL LIVE.*

www.ingramcontent.com/pod-product-compliance
Lightning Source LLC
LaVergne TN
LVHW100315210926
848480LV00003B/1138
9781940461311